Copyright ©2020 Arnold Kunitz Ph.D

All rights reserved. No part of this publication may be reproduced, distributed, or transmitted in any form or by any means, including photocopying, recording, or other electronic or mechanical methods, without the prior written permission of the publisher, except in the case of brief quotations embodied in critical reviews and certain other noncommercial uses permitted by copyright law.

CONTENTS

Introduction
What is sleep apnea?
  Types of sleep apnea
  Diagnosis
  Tests
  Therapies
  Surgery or other procedures
  Central sleep apnea
    Symptoms
    When to see a doctor
    Causes
    Risk factors
    Complications
  Complex sleep apnea
    Prevalence
    How common is complex sleep apnea?
    Causes
    Effects and Treatment
Signs of sleep apnea
Major warning signs
  Other warning signs
Who gets sleep apnea?

What causes sleep apnea?
What are the symptoms of sleep apnea?
How is sleep apnea diagnosed?
What are the treatments for sleep apnea?
Coping with Sleep Apnea
6 Lifestyle Remedies for Sleep Apnea
Myths and Facts About Sleep Apnea
- Sleep Apnea Is Just Snoring
- Sleep Apnea Is No Big Deal
- It Blocks Your Breathing
- Only Older People Get It
- Alcohol Will Help You Sleep
- Sleep Apnea Is Rare in Kids
- Losing Weight Can Help
- A Mouthpiece Might Work, Too
- CPAP Is an Effective Treatment
- Surgery Is the Surest Way to Fix Apnea

Conclusion

INTRODUCTION

Sleep apnea is a sleeping disorder that can lead to serious health problems, such as high blood pressure and heart trouble, if untreated. Untreated sleep apnea causes breathing to stop repeatedly during sleep, causing loud snoring and daytime tiredness, even with a full night's sleep. Sleep apnea can affect anyone, but most often older men who are overweight.

WHAT IS SLEEP APNEA?

Many people treat snoring as a joke or something to feel embarrassed about. But loud snoring especially when accompanied by daytime fatigue may be a sign of sleep apnea, a common but serious disorder in which breathing repeatedly stops and starts as you sleep. If you have sleep apnea, you're probably not aware of these short breathing pauses that occur hundreds of times a night, jolting you out of your natural sleep rhythm. All you know is that you don't feel as energetic, mentally sharp, or productive during the day as you should.

The most common type of sleep apnea obstructive sleep apnea occurs when the airway is blocked, causing pauses in breathing and loud snoring. Since sleep apnea only occurs while you're sleeping, you may only discover you have a problem when a bed partner or roommate complains about your snoring. Though you may feel self-conscious about it or tempted to just make light of your snoring, it's something you shouldn't ignore. Sleep apnea can take a serious toll on your physical and emotional health.

The chronic sleep deprivation caused by sleep apnea can result in daytime sleepiness, slow reflexes, poor concentration, and an increased risk of accidents. Sleep apnea can cause moodiness, irritability, and even lead to depression.

It can also result in other serious physical health problems such as diabetes, heart disease, liver problems, and weight gain. With the right treatment and self-help strategies, however, you can control your snoring and the symptoms of sleep apnea, get your sleep back on track, and feel refreshed and alert during the day.

TYPES OF SLEEP APNEA

Obstructive sleep apnea is the most common type of sleep apnea. It occurs when the soft tissue in the back of the throat relaxes during sleep and blocks the airway, often causing you to snore loudly.

Central sleep apnea is a much less common type of sleep apnea that involves the central nervous system, occurring when the brain fails to signal the muscles that control breathing. People with central sleep apnea seldom snore.

Complex sleep apnea is a combination of obstructive sleep apnea and central sleep apnea.

DIAGNOSIS

To diagnose your condition, your doctor may make an evaluation based on your signs and symptoms, an examination, and tests. Your doctor may refer you to a sleep specialist in a sleep center for further evaluation.

You'll have a physical examination, and your doctor will examine the back of your throat, mouth and nose for extra tissue or abnormalities. Your doctor may measure your neck and waist circumference and check your blood pressure.

A sleep specialist may conduct additional evaluations to diagnose your condition, determine the severity of your condition and plan your treatment. The evaluation may involve overnight monitoring of your breathing and other body functions as you sleep.

TESTS

Tests to detect obstructive sleep apnea include:
Polysomnography. During this sleep study, you're hooked up to equipment that monitors your heart, lung and brain activity, breathing patterns, arm and leg movements, and blood oxygen levels while you sleep. You may have a full night study, in which you're monitored all night, or a split night sleep study.

In a split night sleep study, you'll be monitored during the first half of the night. If you're diagnosed with obstructive sleep apnea, staff may wake you and give you continuous positive airway pressure for the second half of the night. Polysomnography can help your doctor diagnose obstructive sleep apnea and adjust positive airway pressure therapy, if appropriate.

This sleep study can also help rule out other sleep disorders that can cause excessive daytime sleepiness but require different treatments, such as leg movements during sleep (periodic limb movements) or sudden bouts of sleep during the day (narcolepsy).

Home sleep apnea testing. Under certain circumstances, your doctor may provide you with an atom version of polysomnography to diagnose obstructive sleep apnea. This test usually involves measurement of airflow, breathing patterns and blood oxygen levels, and possibly limb movements and snoring intensity.

Your doctor also may refer you to an ear, nose and throat doctor to rule out any anatomic blockage in your nose or throat.

THERAPIES

Continuous positive airway pressure (CPAP) mask

Positive airway pressure. If you have obstructive sleep apnea, you may benefit from positive airway pressure. In this treatment, a machine delivers air pressure through a piece that fits into your nose or is placed over your nose and mouth while you sleep. Positive airway pressure reduces the number of respiratory events that occur as you sleep, reduces daytime sleepiness and improves your quality of life.

The most common type is called continuous positive airway pressure, or CPAP. With this treatment, the pressure of the air breathed is continuous, constant and somewhat greater than that of the surrounding air, which is just enough to keep your upper airway passages open. This air pressure prevents obstructive sleep apnea and snoring.

Although CPAP is the most consistently successful and most commonly used method of treating obstructive sleep apnea, some people find the mask cumbersome, uncomfortable or loud. However, newer machines are smaller and less noisy than older machines and there are a variety of mask designs for individual comfort. Also, with some practice, most people learn to adjust the mask to obtain a comfortable and secure fit. You may need to try different types to find a suitable mask. Several options are available, such as nasal masks, nasal pillows or face masks.

If you're having particular difficulties tolerating pressure, some machines have special adaptive pressure functions to improve comfort. You also may benefit from using a humidifier along with your CPAP system. CPAP may be given at a continuous (fixed) pressure or varied (autotitrating) pressure. In fixed CPAP, the pressure stays constant. In autotitrating CPAP, the levels of pressure are adjusted if the device senses increased airway resistance.

Bilevel positive airway pressure (BPAP), another type of positive airway pressure, delivers a preset amount of pressure when you breathe in and a different amount of pressure when you breathe out. CPAP is more commonly used because it's been well studied for obstructive sleep apnea and has been shown to effectively treat obstructive sleep apnea. However, for people who have difficulty tolerating fixed CPAP, BPAP or autotitrating CPAP may be worth a try.

Don't stop using your positive airway pressure machine if you have problems. Check with your doctor to see what adjustments you can make to improve its comfort.

In addition, contact your doctor if you still snore despite treatment, if you begin snoring again or if your weight goes up or down by 10% or more.

Mouthpiece (oral device). Though positive airway pressure is often an effective treatment, oral appliances are an alternative for some people with mild or moderate obstructive sleep apnea. These devices may reduce your sleepiness and improve your quality of life. These devices are designed to keep your throat open. Some devices keep your airway open by bringing your lower jaw forward, which can sometimes relieve snoring and obstructive sleep apnea. Other devices hold your tongue in a different position.

If you and your doctor decide to explore this option, you'll need to see a dentist experienced in dental sleep medicine appliances for the fitting and follow-up therapy. A number of devices are available. Close follow-up is needed to ensure successful treatment.

SURGERY OR OTHER PROCEDURES

Surgery is usually considered only if other therapies haven't been effective or haven't been appropriate options for you. Surgical options may include:

Surgical removal of tissue. Uvulopalatopharyngoplasty (UPPP) is a procedure in which your doctor removes tissue from the back of your mouth and top of your throat. Your tonsils and adenoids may be removed as well. UPPP usually is performed in a hospital and requires a general anesthetic.

Doctors sometimes remove tissue from the back of the throat with a laser (laser assisted uvulopalatoplasty) or with radiofrequency energy (radiofrequency ablation) to treat snoring. These procedures don't treat obstructive sleep apnea, but they may reduce snoring.

Upper airway stimulation. This new device is approved for use in people with moderate to severe obstructive sleep apnea who can't tolerate CPAP or BPAP. A small, thin impulse generator (hypoglossal nerve stimulator) is implanted under the skin in the upper chest. The device detects your breathing patterns and, when necessary, stimulates the nerve that controls movement of the tongue.

Studies have found that upper airway stimulation leads to significant improvement in obstructive sleep apnea symptoms and improvements in quality of life.

Jaw surgery (maxillomandibular advancement). In this procedure, the upper and lower parts of your jaw are moved forward from the rest of your facial bones. This enlarges the space behind the tongue and soft palate, making obstruction less likely. Surgical opening in the neck (tracheostomy). You may need this form of surgery if other treatments have failed and you have severe, life-threatening obstructive sleep apnea.

During a tracheostomy, your surgeon makes an opening in your neck and inserts a metal or plastic tube through which you breathe. Air passes in and out of your lungs, bypassing the blocked air passage in your throat.

Implants. This minimally invasive treatment involves placement of three tiny polyester rods in the soft palate. These inserts stiffen and support the tissue of the soft palate and reduce upper airway collapse and snoring. This treatment is recommended only for people with mild obstructive sleep apnea.

Other types of surgery may help reduce snoring and sleep apnea by clearing or enlarging air passages, including:

Nasal surgery to remove polyps or straighten a crooked partition between your nostrils (deviated septum)

Surgery to remove enlarged tonsils or adenoids.

CENTRAL SLEEP APNEA

Central sleep apnea is a disorder in which your breathing repeatedly stops and starts during sleep. Central sleep apnea occurs because your brain doesn't send proper signals to the muscles that control your breathing. This condition is different from obstructive sleep apnea; in which you can't breathe normally because of upper airway obstruction. Central sleep apnea is less common than obstructive sleep apnea.

Central sleep apnea may occur as a result of other conditions, such as heart failure and stroke. Sleeping at a high altitude also may cause central sleep apnea.

Treatments for central sleep apnea may involve treating existing conditions, using a device to assist breathing or using supplemental oxygen.

SYMPTOMS

Common signs and symptoms of central sleep apnea include:

Observed episodes of stopped breathing or abnormal breathing patterns during sleep

Abrupt awakenings accompanied by shortness of breath

Shortness of breath that's relieved by sitting up

Difficulty staying asleep (insomnia)

Excessive daytime sleepiness (hypersomnia)

Chest pain at night

Difficulty concentrating

Mood changes

Morning headaches

Snoring

Lower tolerance for exercise

Although snoring indicates some degree of airflow obstruction, snoring also may be heard in the presence of central sleep apnea. However, snoring may not be as prominent with central sleep apnea as it is with obstructive sleep apnea.

WHEN TO SEE A DOCTOR

Consult a medical professional if you experience or if your partner observes any signs or symptoms of central sleep apnea, particularly the following:

Shortness of breath that awakens you from sleep

Intermittent pauses in your breathing during sleep

Difficulty staying asleep

Excessive daytime drowsiness, which may cause you to fall asleep while you're working, watching television or even driving

Ask your doctor about any sleep problem that leaves you chronically fatigued, sleepy and irritable. Excessive daytime drowsiness may be due to other disorders, such as not allowing yourself time to get enough sleep at night (chronic sleep deprivation), sudden attacks of sleep (narcolepsy) or obstructive sleep apnea.

CAUSES

Central sleep apnea occurs when your brain fails to transmit signals to your breathing muscles. Central sleep apnea can be caused by a number of conditions that affect the ability of your brainstem which links your brain to your spinal cord and controls many functions such as heart rate and breathing to control your breathing.

The cause varies with the type of central sleep apnea you have.
Types include:
Cheyne Stokes breathing. This type of central sleep apnea is most commonly associated with congestive heart failure or stroke. Cheyne Stokes breathing is characterized by a gradual increase and then decrease in breathing effort and airflow. During the weakest breathing effort, a total lack of airflow (central sleep apnea) can occur.

Drug induced apnea. Taking certain medications such as opioids — including morphine (Ms Contin, Kadian, others), oxycodone (Roxicodone, Oxycontin, others) or codeine — may cause your breathing to become irregular, to increase and decrease in a regular pattern, or to temporarily stop completely.

High altitude periodic breathing. A Cheyne Stokes breathing pattern may occur if you're exposed to a very high altitude. The change in oxygen at this altitude is the reason for the alternating rapid breathing (hyperventilation) and under breathing.

Treatment emergent central sleep apnea. Some people with obstructive sleep apnea develop central sleep apnea while using continuous positive airway pressure (CPAP) for their sleep apnea treatment. This condition is known as treatment emergent central sleep apnea and is a combination of obstructive and central sleep apneas.

Medical condition induced central sleep apnea. Several medical conditions, including end stage kidney disease and stroke, may give rise to central sleep apnea of the non Cheyne Stokes variety.

Idiopathic (primary) central sleep apnea. The cause of this uncommon type of central sleep apnea isn't known.

RISK FACTORS

Certain factors put you at increased risk of central sleep apnea:

Sex: Males are more likely to develop central sleep apnea than are females.

Age: Central sleep apnea is more common among older adults, especially adults older than age 65, possibly because they may have other medical conditions or sleep patterns that are more likely to cause central sleep apnea.

Heart disorders: People with irregular heartbeats (atrial fibrillation) or whose heart muscles don't pump enough blood for the body's needs (congestive heart failure) are at greater risk of central sleep apnea.

Stroke, brain tumor or a structural brainstem lesion. These brain conditions can impair the brain's ability to regulate breathing.

High altitude: Sleeping at an altitude higher than you're accustomed to may increase your risk of sleep apnea. High altitude sleep apnea is no longer a problem a few weeks after returning to a lower altitude.

Opioid use: Opioid medications may increase the risk of central sleep apnea.

CPAP: Some people with obstructive sleep apnea develop central sleep apnea while using continuous positive airway pressure (CPAP). This condition is known as treatment emergent central sleep apnea. It is a combination of obstructive and central sleep apneas.

For most people, treatment emergent central sleep apnea goes away with continued use of a CPAP device. Other people may be treated with a different kind of positive airway pressure therapy.

COMPLICATIONS

Central sleep apnea is a serious medical condition. Some complications include:

Fatigue. The repeated awakenings associated with sleep apnea make normal, restorative sleep impossible. People with central sleep apnea often experience severe fatigue, daytime drowsiness and irritability.

You may have difficulty concentrating and find yourself falling asleep at work, while watching television or even when driving.

Cardiovascular problems. In addition, sudden drops in blood oxygen levels that occur during central sleep apnea may adversely affect heart health. If there's underlying heart disease, these repeated multiple episodes of low blood oxygen (hypoxia or hypoxemia) worsen prognosis and increase the risk of abnormal heart rhythms.

COMPLEX SLEEP APNEA

First, obstructive sleep apnea2 occurs when the upper airway (or throat) collapses during sleep. This can trigger drops in the blood's oxygen levels as well as arousals, or awakenings from sleep. Based on a diagnostic sleep study called a polysomnogram, this condition is present when there are five or more obstructive events occurring per hour of sleep. These airway collapses may go by various names, including obstructive apneas, mixed apneas, hypopneas, and respiratory related arousals (RERAs).

Once obstructive sleep apnea is identified, the most common and effective treatment is the use of CPAP therapy. This treatment delivers a constant flow of air through a facial mask. This additional air keeps the airway from collapsing, or obstructing, and also resolves snoring. In some cases, it may trigger changes in breathing that result in breath holding, a condition called central sleep apnea.

By definition, complex sleep apnea occurs with the use of CPAP treatment. Obstructive events resolve with therapy, while central apnea events emerge or persist with therapy. These central apnea events must occur at least five times per hour and they should constitute more than 50% of the total number of apnea and hypopnea events. Therefore, if you have a total of 100 apnea events noted while using CPAP therapy, and only 49 (or more likely fewer) are central apnea events, you do not have complex sleep apnea. It is very common for some central apnea events to emerge, but they may not require any additional intervention beyond time.

PREVALENCE

Complex sleep apnea may be relatively common during the initial treatment period with CPAP or even bi-level therapy. These central apnea events are not better explained by the use of medications (like narcotics or opioid pain medicines) and are not due to heart failure or stroke. There may be a high number of arousals from sleep and each awakening may be followed by an episode of post arousal central sleep apnea. These events are more commonly seen in non REM sleep and may improve slightly in stage 3 or slow wave sleep.

HOW COMMON IS COMPLEX SLEEP APNEA?

This is actually a difficult question to answer. The true incidence and degree of persistence are not well defined, due to the fact that it often variably resolves as PAP therapy continues. It is estimated to affect from 2% to 20% of people as they start using CPAP therapy and may be seen more often in the first or second night of use. Therefore, it may be over identified as part of a titration study in a sleep center. Fortunately, it only persists with therapy in about 2% of people.

CAUSES

The exact causes of complex sleep apnea are not fully understood. There may be a number of contributions to the condition, and not all are due to CPAP therapy. Some individuals may be predisposed towards the condition due to instability in their control of breathing. It may occur more commonly among those with difficulty maintaining sleep, such as with insomnia. It seems to be triggered by low carbon dioxide levels in some. If someone has more severe sleep apnea initially (with a higher apneahypopnea index,6 or AHI) or has more central apnea events noted prior to treatment, this may increase the risk. It also seems to occur more in men.

It is interesting to note that other treatments of sleep apnea also seem to increase the risk of developing complex sleep apnea. Surgery and the use of an oral appliance have both been reported to trigger central sleep apnea. It may also occur if the pressures of the PAP therapy are either too high or conversely too low, as set during a titration study or in subsequent home use.

EFFECTS AND TREATMENT

Even though complex sleep apnea generally resolves over time, there are still 2% of people in whom the condition persists and there may be other consequences. Some of these people may require alternative treatments to resolve the disorder.

Complex sleep apnea may be noted to persist on routine download of PAP compliance data. This will usually occur at a routine follow up appointment with your sleep specialist in the first 3 months of use. If more than five central apnea events are occurring per hour, despite the obstructive sleep apnea events resolving, this might prompt changes. Why might this matter?

Persistent complex sleep apnea associated with a high residual AHI may cause continued sleep fragmentation and oxygen desaturation. This may lead to daytime sleepiness and other long-term health effects. Importantly, this may also compromise PAP therapy: the user may report little benefit and have poor long-term adherence to the treatment.

It is important to recognize that there may be night to night variability. In the context of your initial condition, some elevations in the AHI may be tolerated if the overall response to therapy is favorable. Though the devices can provide a rough measure of central apnea events, these are not perfect, and this may be better assessed via a standard polysomnogram.

Resolution of complex sleep apnea may depend on addressing the underlying causes. For example, if the pressures used are simply too high (or, less often, too low), a simple adjustment may resolve the matter. If awakenings are occurring due to mask leak, a proper fitting may help. In some cases, it may be necessary to switch to bi-level ST (with a timed breath rate that can be delivered during breath pauses) or ASV therapy. These therapy modalities will often require a titration study to find the optimal device settings.

The most prudent treatment is often the most effective: time. Complex sleep apnea will usually improve in 98% of cases as therapy continues. It may not require any further intervention beyond waiting and watching the remaining events resolve on their own.

SIGNS OF SLEEP APNEA

It can be tough to identify sleep apnea on your own, since the most prominent symptoms only occur when you're asleep. But you can get around this difficulty by asking a bed partner to observe your sleep habits, or by recording yourself during sleep. If pauses occur while you snore, and if choking or gasping follows the pauses, these are major warning signs that you have sleep apnea.

MAJOR WARNING SIGNS

Loud and chronic snoring almost every night

Choking, snorting, or gasping during sleep

Pauses in breathing

Waking up at night feeling short of breath

Daytime sleepiness and fatigue, no matter how much time you spend in bed

OTHER WARNING SIGNS

Waking up with a dry mouth or sore throat

Insomnia or nighttime awakenings; restless or fitful sleep

Going to the bathroom frequently during the night

Forgetfulness and difficulty concentrating

Uncharacteristic moodiness, irritability, or depression

Morning headaches

Impotence

WHO GETS SLEEP APNEA?

Sleep apnea occurs in about 25% of men and nearly 10% of women. Sleep apnea can affect people of all ages, including babies and children and particularly people over the age of 50 and those who are overweight.

Certain physical traits and clinical features are common in patients with obstructive sleep apnea. These include excessive weight, large neck and structural abnormalities reducing the diameter of the upper airway, such as nasal obstruction, a low hanging soft palate, enlarged tonsils or a small jaw with an overbite.

WHAT CAUSES SLEEP APNEA?

Obstructive sleep apnea is caused by a blockage of the airway, usually when the soft tissue in the rear of the throat collapses during sleep. Central sleep apnea is usually observed in patients with central nervous system dysfunction, such as following a stroke or in patients with neuromuscular diseases like amyotrophic lateral sclerosis (ALS, Lou Gehrig's disease). It is also common in patients with heart failure and other forms of heart, kidney or lung disease.

Various factors can contribute to the blocking or collapse of the airway:

Muscular changes: When people sleep, the muscles that keep the airway open relax, along with the tongue, causing the airway to narrow. Normally, this relaxation does not prevent the flow of air in and out of the lungs, but in sleep apnea, it can.

Physical obstructions: Additional thickened tissue or excessive fat stores around the airway can restrict the airflow, and any air that squeezes past can cause the loud snoring typically associated with OSA.

Brain function: In central sleep apnea (CSA), the neurological controls for breathing are faulty, causing the control and rhythm of breathing to malfunction. CSA is usually associated with an underlying medical condition, such as a stroke or heart failure, recent ascent to high altitude, or the use of pain relief medication.

When the airway becomes completely blocked, the snoring stops and there is no breathing for a 1020 second time period or until the brain senses the apnea and signals the muscles to tighten, returning the airflow. This pause in breathing is known as apnea.

Although this process continues hundreds of times throughout the night, the individual experiencing the apnea is not conscious of the problem.

WHAT ARE THE SYMPTOMS OF SLEEP APNEA?

Often the first signs of OSA are recognized not by the patient, but by the bed partner. Many of those affected have no sleep complaints. The most common signs and symptoms of OSA include:

Snoring.

Daytime sleepiness or fatigue.

Restlessness during sleep, frequent nighttime awakenings.

Sudden awakenings with a sensation of gasping or choking.

Dry mouth or sore throat upon awakening.

Cognitive impairment, such as trouble concentrating, forgetfulness or irritability.

Mood disturbances (depression or anxiety).

Night sweats.

Frequent nighttime urination.

Sexual dysfunction.

Headaches.

People with central sleep apnea more often report recurrent awakenings or insomnia, although they may also experience a choking or gasping sensation upon awakening.

Symptoms in children may not be as obvious and include:
Poor school performance.

Sluggishness or sleepiness, often misinterpreted as laziness in the classroom.

Daytime mouth breathing and swallowing difficulty.

Inward movement of the ribcage when inhaling.

Unusual sleeping positions, such as sleeping on the hands and knees, or with the neck hyperextended.

Excessive sweating at night.

Learning and behavioral disorders (hyperactivity, attention deficits).

Bedwetting.

HOW IS SLEEP APNEA DIAGNOSED?

If your doctor determines that you have symptoms suggestive of sleep apnea, you may be asked to have a sleep evaluation with a sleep specialist or may order an overnight sleep study to objectively evaluate for sleep apnea.

Testing includes an overnight sleep study called a polysomnogram (PSG). A PSG is performed in a sleep laboratory under the direct supervision of a trained technologist. During the test, a variety of body functions, such as the electrical activity of the brain, eye movements, muscle activity, heart rate, breathing patterns, air flow, and blood oxygen levels are recorded at night during sleep. After the study is completed, the number of times breathing is impaired during sleep is tallied and the severity of the sleep apnea is graded.

For adults, a Home Sleep Test (HST) can sometimes be performed instead. This is a modified type of sleep study that can be done in the comfort of home. It records fewer body functions than PSG, including airflow, breathing effort, blood oxygen levels and snoring to confirm a diagnosis of moderate to severe obstructive sleep apnea.

An HST is not appropriate to be used as a screening tool

for patients without symptoms. It's not used for patients with significant medical problems (such as heart failure, moderate to severe cardiac disease, neuromuscular disease or moderate to severe pulmonary disease). It's also not used for patients who have other sleep disorders (such as central sleep apnea, restless legs syndrome, insomnia, circadian rhythm disorders, parasomnias or narcolepsy) in addition to the suspected obstructive sleep apnea.

Option 1: CPAP
Continuous Positive Airflow Pressure (CPAP) is the most common treatment for moderate to severe obstructive sleep apnea. The CPAP device is a masklike machine that covers your nose and mouth, providing a constant stream of air that keeps your breathing passages open while you sleep.

If you've given up on sleep apnea machines in the past because of discomfort, you owe it to yourself to give them a second look. CPAP technology is constantly being updated and improved, and the new CPAP devices are lighter, quieter, and more comfortable. In many cases, you'll experience immediate symptom relief and a huge boost in your mental and physical energy.

Option 2: Other breathing devices
In addition to CPAP, there are other devices that a sleep specialist may recommend for sleep apnea treatment:

Expiratory positive airway pressure (EPAP) single use devices fit over the nostrils to help keep the airway open and are smaller, less intrusive than CPAP machines. These may benefit people with mild to moderate obstructive sleep apnea.

Bilevel positive airway pressure (BiPAP or BPAP) devices can be used for those who are unable to adapt to using CPAP, or for central sleep apnea sufferers who need assistance for a weak breathing pattern. This device automatically adjusts the pressure while you're sleeping, providing more pressure when you inhale, less when you exhale. Some BiPAP devices also automatically deliver a breath if the mask detects that you haven't taken one for a certain number of seconds.

Adaptive servoventilation (ASV) devices can be used for treating central sleep apnea as well as obstructive sleep apnea. The ASV device stores information about your normal breathing pattern and automatically uses airflow pressure to prevent pauses in your breathing while you're asleep.

Option 3: Oral appliances
Custommade oral appliances are becoming an increasingly popular means of treatment as they offer numerous advantages over breathing devices. They're quieter, more portable, and tend to be more comfortable. While there are many different oral appliances approved for sleep apnea treatment, most are either acrylic devices that fit inside your mouth, much like an athletic mouth guard, or fit around your head and chin to adjust the position of your lower jaw.

Two common oral devices are the mandibular advancement device and the tongue retaining device. These devices open your airway by bringing your lower jaw or your tongue forward during sleep.

Since there are so many different devices available, it

may take some experimentation to find the appliance that works best for you. It's also very important to get fitted by a dentist specializing in sleep apnea, and to see the dentist on a regular basis to monitor any problems and periodically adjust the mouthpiece. There are some potential side effects to oral appliances, including soreness, saliva buildup, and damage or permanent change in position of the jaw, teeth, and mouth. These could be more serious in poorly fitted devices.

Option 4: Sleep apnea implants
One of the newest treatments for sleep apnea involves the insertion of a pacemaker system that stimulates muscles to keep airways open so you can breathe during sleep. The new treatment has been approved by the FDA in the U.S. for people with moderate to severe obstructive sleep apnea.

Although the technology is relatively new (and expensive), studies suggest it may also benefit people with central sleep apnea.

Option 5: Surgery
If you have exhausted other sleep apnea treatment options, surgery can increase the size of your airway, thus reducing episodes of sleep apnea.

The surgeon may remove tonsils, adenoids, or excess tissue at the back of the throat or inside the nose, reconstruct the jaw to enlarge the upper airway, or implant plastic rods into the soft palate. Surgery carries risks of complications and infections, and in some rare cases, symptoms can become worse after surgery.

WHAT ARE THE TREATMENTS FOR SLEEP APNEA?

Conservative treatments: In mild cases of obstructive sleep apnea, conservative therapy may be all that is needed.

1. Overweight persons can benefit from losing weight. Even a 10% weight loss can reduce the number of apneic events for most patients. However, losing weight can be difficult to do with untreated obstructive sleep apnea due to increased appetite and metabolism changes that can happen with obstructive sleep apnea.

2. Individuals with obstructive sleep apnea should avoid the use of alcohol and certain sleeping pills, which make the airway more likely to collapse during sleep and prolong the apneic periods.

3. In some patients with mild obstructive sleep apnea, breathing pauses occur only when they sleep on their backs. In such cases, using a wedge pillow or other devices that help them sleep in a side position may help.

4. People with sinus problems or nasal congestion should use nasal sprays or breathing strips to reduce snoring and improve airflow for more comfortable nighttime

breathing. Avoiding sleep deprivation is important for all patients with sleep disorders.

Mechanical therapy: Positive Airway Pressure (PAP) therapy is the preferred initial treatment for most people with obstructive sleep apnea. With PAP therapy, patients wear a mask over their nose and/or mouth. An air blower gently forces air through the nose and/or mouth. The air pressure is adjusted so that it is just enough to prevent the upper airway tissues from collapsing during sleep. PAP therapy prevents airway closure while in use, but apnea episodes return when PAP is stopped or if it is used improperly. There are several styles, and types of positive airway pressure devices depending on specific needs of patients. Styles and types include:

CPAP (Continuous Positive Airway Pressure) is the most widely used of the PAP devices. The machine is set at one single pressure. BiLevel PAP uses one pressure during inhalation (breathing in), and a lower pressure during exhalation (breathing out). There is a criterion that must be met before health insurance will cover the bilevel. This usually means that the CPAP machine must be tried first with no success and these results documented before insurance will pay for a bilevel.

Auto CPAP or Auto BiLevel PAP uses a range of pressures that selfregulates during use depending on pressure requirements detected by the machine. Adaptive ServoVentilation (ASV) is a type of noninvasive ventilation that is used for patients with central sleep apnea, which acts to keep the airway open and delivers a mandatory breath when needed.

Mandibular advancement devices: These are devices for patients with mild to moderate obstructive sleep apnea. Dental appliances or oral mandibular advancement devices that help to prevent the tongue from blocking the throat and/or advance the lower jaw forward can be made. These devices help keep the airway open during sleep. A sleep specialist and dentist (with expertise in oral appliances for this purpose) should jointly determine if this treatment is best for you.

Hypoglossal nerve stimulator: A stimulator is implanted under the skin on the right side of the chest with electrodes tunneled under the skin to the hypoglossal nerve in the neck and to intercostal muscles (between two ribs) in the chest. The device is turned on at bedtime with a remote control. With each breath, the hypoglossal nerve is stimulated, the tongue moves forward out of the airway and the airway is opened.

Surgery: Surgical procedures may help people with obstructive sleep apnea and others who snore but don't have sleep apnea. Among the many types of surgeries done are outpatient procedures. Surgery is for people who have excessive or malformed tissue obstructing airflow through the nose or throat, such as a deviated nasal septum, markedly enlarged tonsils or small lower jaw with an overbite that causes the throat to be abnormally narrow. These procedures are typically performed after sleep apnea has failed to respond to conservative measures and a trial of CPAP.

Types of surgery include:
Somnoplasty: is a minimally invasive procedure that uses radiofrequency energy to reduce the soft tissue in the upper airway.

Tonsillectomy: is a procedure that removes the tonsillar tissue in the back of the throat which is a common cause of obstruction in children with sleep apnea.

Uvulopalatopharyngoplasty (UPPP): is a procedure that removes soft tissue on the back of the throat and palate, increasing the width of the airway at the throat opening.

Mandibular/maxillary advancement surgery: is a surgical correction of certain facial abnormalities or throat obstructions that contribute to obstructive sleep apnea. This is an invasive procedure that is reserved for patients with severe obstructive sleep apnea with head face abnormalities. Nasal surgery includes correction of nasal obstructions, such as a deviated septum.

COPING WITH SLEEP APNEA

The most important part of treatment for people with OSA is using the CPAP whenever they sleep. The health benefits of this therapy can be enormous, but only if used correctly. If you are having problems adjusting your CPAP or you're experiencing side effects of wearing the appliance, talk to the doctor who prescribed it and ask for assistance.

Getting adequate sleep is essential to maintaining health in OSA patients. If you have symptoms of insomnia such as difficulty falling asleep, staying asleep, or waking up unrefreshed, talk to your doctor about treatment options. Keep in mind that certain store purchased and prescription sleep aids may impair breathing in OSA patients. One exception is ramelteon, which was studied in mild and moderate OSA patients and found to not harm their breathing.

6 LIFESTYLE REMEDIES FOR SLEEP APNEA

Sleep apnea lifestyle remedies

Traditional treatments for sleep apnea include wearing a CPAP mask at night. Though effective, some people find this method uncomfortable. Some home remedies may offer the same benefits. Here are six alternative treatments to reduce sleep apnea symptoms.

1. Maintain a healthy weight

Doctors commonly recommend people with sleep apnea to lose weight. Obesity, specifically in the upper body, can increase the risk of airway obstruction and narrow nasal passages. These obstructions can cause you to stop breathing suddenly or for lengths of time while sleeping.

Maintaining a healthy weight can keep your airways clear and reduce sleep apnea symptoms. Research shows that modest weight reduction in people with obesity can eliminate the need for upper airway surgery or long-term CPAP therapy.

In some cases, weight loss can eliminate sleep apnea. However, if you regain the weight, it's possible for the condition to return.

2. Try yoga
Regular exercise can increase your energy level, strengthen your heart, and improve sleep apnea. Yoga can specifically improve your respiratory strength and encourage oxygen flow.

Sleep apnea is associated with decreased oxygen saturation in your blood. Yoga can improve your oxygen levels through its various breathing exercises. As a result, yoga reduces the amount of sleep interruptions you may experience.

3. Alter your sleep position
Though a small change, altering your sleep position can reduce sleep apnea symptoms and improve your night's rest. A 2006 study found that more than half of obstructive sleep apnea cases are dependent on position.

Studies have shown sleeping on your back called the supine position can worsen symptoms. For some adults, sleeping on the side can help breathing return to normal.

However, a 2002 study found that children with sleep apnea sleep better on their backs. Discuss body positioning and your sleep apnea symptoms with your doctor to evaluate your options for treatment.

4. Use a humidifier
Humidifiers are devices that add moisture to the air. Dry air can irritate the body and the respiratory system. Using a humidifier can open your airways, decrease congestion, and encourage clearer breathing.

For added benefits, consider adding lavender, peppermint, or eucalyptus oil to a humidifier. These three essential oils have known anti-inflammatory and soothing benefits.

Follow the manufacturer's instructions on cleaning your humidifier. They can harbor molds and bacteria.

Purchase a humidifier online.

5. Avoid alcohol and smoking
Lifestyle changes can improve your health and encourage better sleeping habits. Consider quitting smoking and limiting your alcohol intake to reduce sleep apnea complications.

Alcohol relaxes the throat muscles that control your breathing. This can lead to snoring and an interrupted sleep cycle. It can also lead to inflammation in your airways, blocking your airflow.

Similar to alcohol, tobacco use can also contribute to inflammation and swelling in your airways. This can worsen your snoring and your sleep apnea.

A 2012 study identified smoking as a risk factor for developing sleep apnea. The study noted that people with sleep apnea may have a predisposition to smoking as well, so treating sleep apnea may help in quitting smoking.

6. Use oral appliances
Oral appliances can help with sleep apnea by repositioning your jaw or tongue to keep your airway open while you sleep.

The two major categories are mandibular advancement devices and tongue stabilizing devices. These work by moving your lower jaw or tongue forward to decrease the obstruction in the back of your throat.

These appliances range from low cost, over the counter (OTC) options to devices that are custom fit by a dentist.

The American Academy of Dental Sleep Medicine supports oral appliances as an effective therapy for sleep apnea.

A 2015 guideline recommends oral appliances for people with sleep apnea who can't tolerate a CPAP device. This guideline endorses custom fit appliances over OTC options because they allow for fine-tuned jaw positioning, which will result in better sleep quality.

MYTHS AND FACTS ABOUT SLEEP APNEA

SLEEP APNEA IS JUST SNORING

Myth. Snoring can be a symptom of the sleep disorder, but there's a big difference between the two. People with the condition actually stop breathing up to 400 times throughout the night. These pauses last 10 to 30 seconds, and they're usually followed by a snort when breathing starts again. This breaks your sleep cycle and can leave you tired during the day.

SLEEP APNEA IS NO BIG DEAL

Myth. All those breaks in sleep take a toll on your body and mind. When the condition goes untreated, it's been linked to job related injuries, car accidents, heart attacks, and strokes.

IT BLOCKS YOUR BREATHING

Fact. The most common type of the disorder is obstructive sleep apnea, or OSA. It happens when your tongue, tonsils, or other tissues in the back of the throat block your airway. When you try to breathe in, the air can't get through. Central sleep apnea is less common than OSA. It means the brain doesn't always signal the body to breathe when it should.

ONLY OLDER PEOPLE GET IT

Myth. Doctors estimate that more than 18 million Americans have sleep apnea. It's more common after age 40, but it can affect people of all ages. You're more likely to have the condition if you're overweight, a man, African American, or Latino. The disorder also tends to run in families.

ALCOHOL WILL HELP YOU SLEEP

Myth. A nightcap may make you drowsy, but it won't help you get the quality rest you need. Alcohol relaxes the muscles in the back of your throat. That makes it easier for the airway to become blocked in people with sleep apnea. Sleeping pills have the same effect.

SLEEP APNEA IS RARE IN KIDS

Myth. OSA is common in children, affecting as many as 1 in 10. In most cases, the symptoms are mild, and the child eventually outgrows it. But some may start to have behavior troubles or serious medical problems because of it.

LOSING WEIGHT CAN HELP

Fact. You can make sleep apnea symptoms better when you shed even a small percentage of your body weight. If you're carrying around extra pounds, talk to your doctor about starting a weight loss program. It also helps to quit smoking, so ask about treatments that can help.

Lying on Your Side Can Help
Fact. If you sleep on your back, gravity can pull the tissues in the throat down, where they're more likely to block your airway. Sleep on your side instead to open your throat. Certain pillows can help keep you on your side. Some people even go to bed in shirts with tennis balls sewn onto the back.

A MOUTHPIECE MIGHT WORK, TOO

Fact. A dentist or orthodontist can fit you with a mouthpiece or oral appliance to ease mild sleep apnea. The device is custom-made for you, and it adjusts the position of your lower jaw and tongue. You put it in at bedtime to help keep your airway open while you sleep.

CPAP IS AN EFFECTIVE TREATMENT

Fact. It stands for continuous positive airway pressure. A CPAP machine blows a steady stream of air into your airway. You can adjust the flow until it's strong enough to keep your airway open while you sleep. It's the most common treatment for adults with moderate to severe OSA.

SURGERY IS THE SUREST WAY TO FIX APNEA

Myth. For some people, an operation may be able to cure OSA. A good example is a child with large tonsils that block her airway. Doctors can remove the tonsils to solve the problem. Some adults can improve their symptoms with surgery to shrink or stiffen floppy tissues. But that's not a good choice for everyone. Talk to your doctor about the pros and cons of an operation before you go that route.

CONCLUSION

Sleep apnea can disrupt your nightly slumber and put you at risk of several serious diseases, but there are ways to control it. Treatments, such as continuous positive airway pressure (CPAP) and oral appliances, help keep oxygen flowing into your lungs while you sleep. Losing weight can also improve sleep apnea symptoms while reducing your heart disease risk.

Printed in Great Britain
by Amazon